#TheKettlebellCleanse

http://workoutkingrule.blogspot.com/

workoutkingrule@gmail.com

Checkout

The Sprint Diet

My Story

If you're looking for a book with perfect spelling, and punctuation than you've come to the wrong place. If you're looking for a book with accurate, and useful information than you've come to the right place.

When I discovered the Kettlebell I was going through a hard time. I had no idea what I was doing. No form of exercise was working for me. I didn't want to go to the gym because I was ashamed of the way I looked. I wanted to do a workout that would preserve my muscle, but would help me lose fat. I started doing research, and by the grace of good luck I ran into the Kettlebell. At first I had no idea what it was or how it worked. I just knew that it was something that I'd seen before in the stores, but I never actually picked it up. I didn't know it came in different sizes. I didn't know what size I needed. All I know is when I started using it my body started to change. At first I didn't know any of the routines or moves. I had no idea you could work out your entire body with it! Little by little I learn different moves, and which muscles they targeted. Little by little I started to discover different combinations of moves that helped me lose weight quickly, and efficiently. Having a kettlebell is like having a gym in your house. People say that the Kettlebell builds muscle, but that depends on how often you up the weight. You have to increase the resistance if you want to increase your muscle size. If you start off with ah 10-pound kettlebell you want to up the weight to 15 or 20. You work towards 30 than you work towards 40, and so on. Don't use a ten-pound kettlebell for three months that's the last thing you want to do! You're not going to see the results you're looking for if you do that. I continued to increase the weight. I continued to increase the complexity of my workouts, and my results shine through.

Throughout my weight-loss journey I would pick things up, and put them down immediately. I didn't feel like anything was working. The Kettlebell is different. For some reason I like doing it. I could feel that it was working for me. I could feel that it was having a positive effect on my body. It wasn't just helping me lose weight it was helping me gain muscle. I could feel muscle growing in me every time I worked out. Above all the kettlebell builds muscle endurance.

I've always had a fear of putting in limitless amounts of work to get no results. It seems like that was always the case with the majority of the workouts I tried. With the Kettlebell what I put in was what I got out that's why I respect it.

The Benefits Of Kettlebell Training

The Kettlebell combines cardio with strength training. I mean drop the mic on stage that's pretty much the greatest benefit of all time. There are very few exercises I can name that actually combine cardio with strength training. Sprinting has the same effect, and guess who has a book on that this guy. It's called The Sprint Diet check it out it's a great read. When you combine cardio, and strength training you get high calorie loss without loss of muscle. Ah hour of kettlebell training can burn 1200 calories that's a lot of calories. Compare that to 500 calories for an hour on the treadmill there's no competition. The

Kettlebell wins hands down! You would have to do almost two, and ah half hours worth of work just to match one hour of kettlebell training. That's not even considering the internal benefits that Kettlebell training has over the treadmill. Even if you consider a more calories aggressive machine like the elliptical you're still only going to get eight maybe 900 calories for an hour. Still no match for the Kettlebell! Not only are you going to burn more calories by using the Kettlebell, but you're also going to build muscle. You're not going to build any muscle on treadmills! It doesn't matter if we're talking about the bike, the elliptical, or even the stair climber the kettlebell's going to win every single time it has no equal. The kettlebell is not nearly as hard as some people make it seem. If you start off slow, and learn the essential exercises it's not hard at all. If anything it can be fun once you become proficient. You want to start off with three basic moves. Once you master them you do more complicated movements. You just need to build up some strength, and some coordination first.

Beginners Moves And Kettlebell Selection

You have to be careful when choosing a kettlebell. You don't want to pick anything that's too heavy. If you do you might throw your back out. This is why it's best to pick your kettlebell in the store. It's easier to shop for a kettlebell online once you've already had some experience with a real kettlebell. Go into the store, and try some moves with some of the kettlebells. See if it feels right. As long as it's not to light it's the right size. If you're a female I suggest you start off with a 10-pound kettlebell. If you're stronger than by all means buy something more advanced. If you're a male I suggest that you start off with a 15 to 20 pound kettlebell. As you become stronger the weight we'll get lighter. At this point you want to up the weight so you can continue gaining muscle. If you keep lifting the same weight you're not going to notice a difference no matter how hard you work! Now that we got that out of the way let's talk about beginner techniques.

First up is *The Kettlebell Swing*. The kettlebell swing is the most popular kettlebell exercise. It works the hips, glutes, hamstrings, lats, ABS, shoulders, chest, and your grip. It's one of the most effective exercises you can do with the Kettlebell. I personally have seen series results from the kettlebell swing. It's my favorite kettlebell move. In the photo you can see exactly how to do a kettlebell swing. As you can see it's all about the hips. When you bring the weight back up the momentum from you thrusting your hips forward is what carries it to the top not your arms. You're thrusting with your hips while squeezing your abs, and your glutes simultaneously. Just make sure you don't let go of the Kettlebell. I did that once and boy did I cause some damage. This exercise makes you so much better at all the other kettlebell moves. It strengthens the key muscles you need to perform more advanced movements.

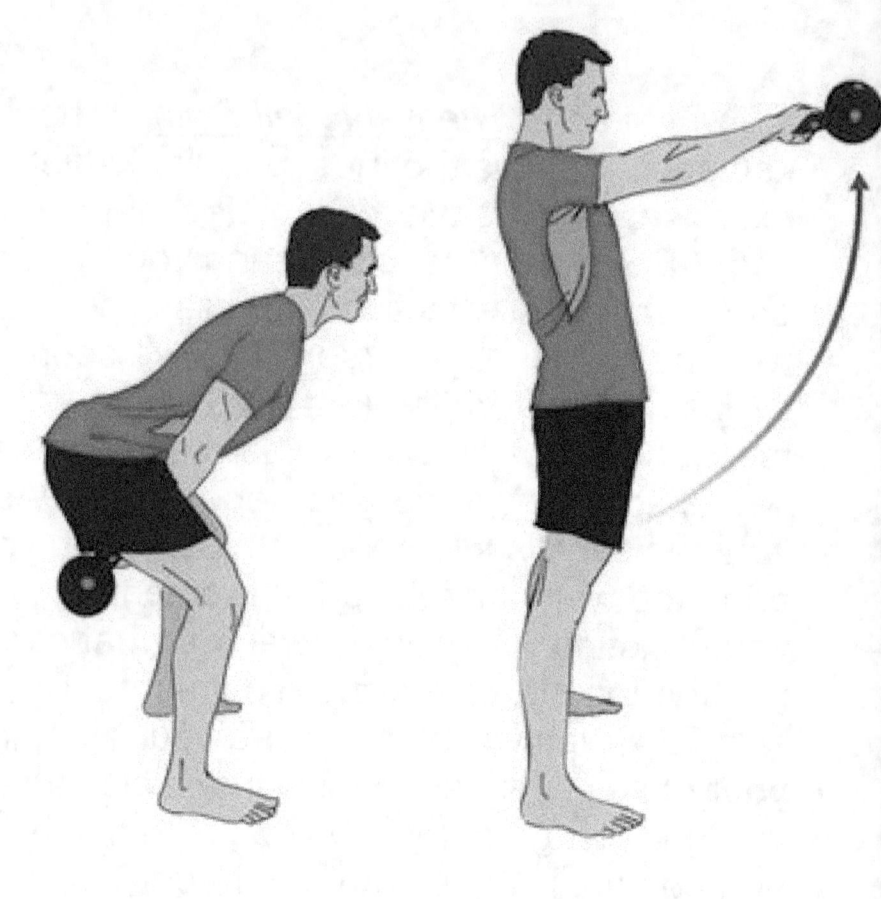

The second move is *The Around The Body Pass*. The around the body pass is the most basic kettlebell move there it's. It's one of the most important moves because it strengthens the core, and the obliques. The kettlebell is a core-blasting beast. Almost every single exercise requires you use your core in some way. The around the body pass strengthens the core, and your oblique's preparing your body to deal with advanced compound movements. The more advanced the move the more it will require core stability. Even though this move looks simple at first you might drop the Kettlebell, I know I did. Passing a heavy weight behind your back might be a little more difficult than you think. Passing the weight behind you forces your core to stabilize your body that's what makes it a key core workout.

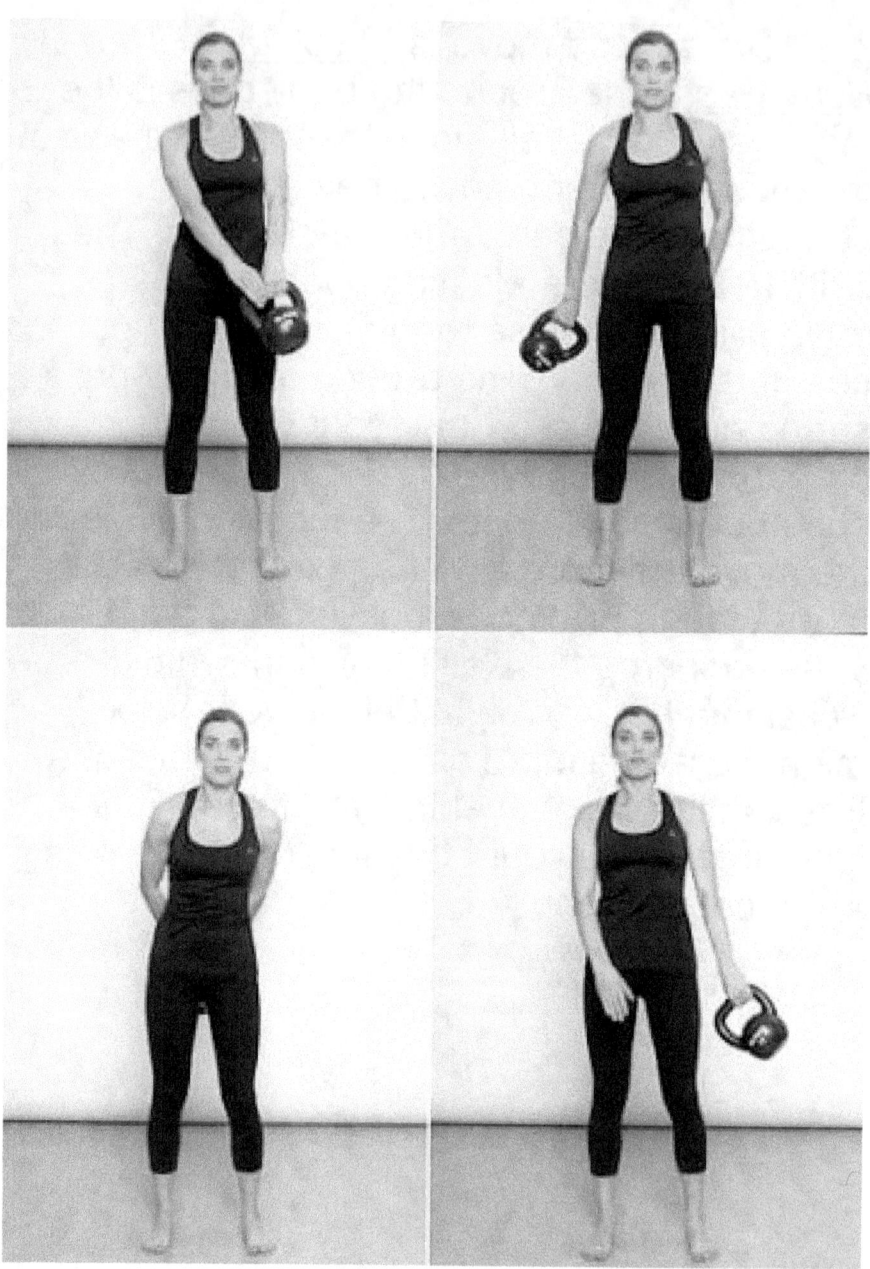

Number three is the _Two Hand Overhead Press_. _The Two Hand Overhead Press_ is a very key beginner moves. It works the shoulders, back, chest, triceps, and the core. These are key muscles that you're going to need throughout any kettlebell routine. Below is a picture of how to perform the _Two Hand Overhead Press_. As you can see it's incredibly simple yet it is incredibly effective.

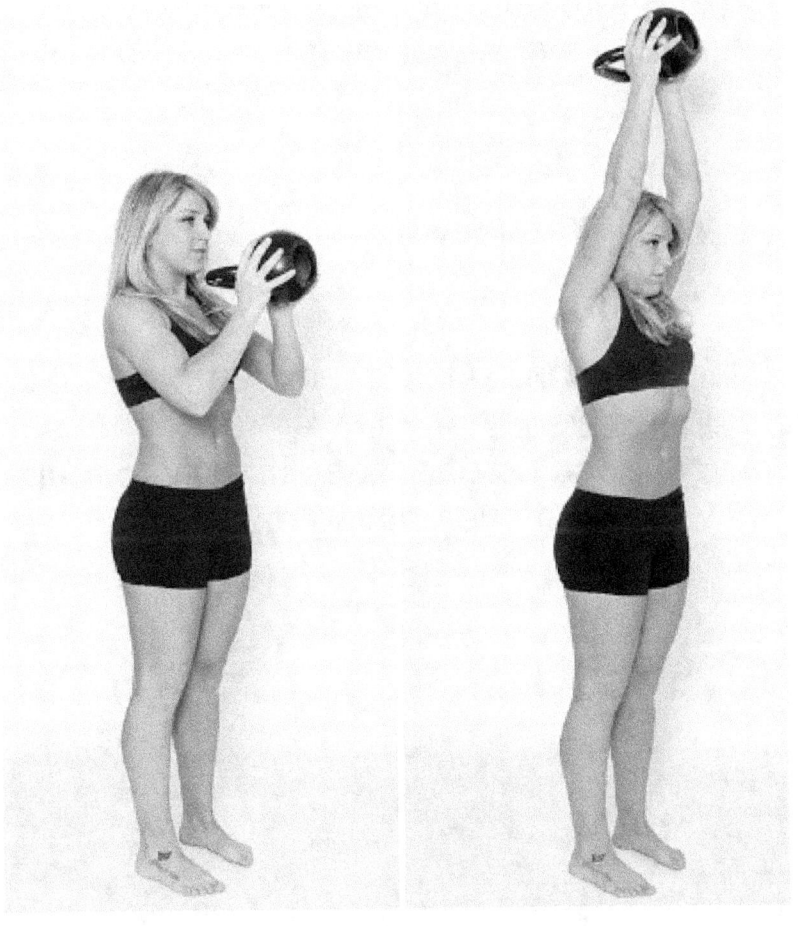

As a beginner workout you would combine all three of these exercises together. You want to do this for a period of at least 30 minutes. A good combination would be 10 minutes of each individual exercise. If that's too boring for you than simply do five minutes of all three two times. Do 30 minutes a day for 15 days, and I guarantee you will notice a difference. In those 15 days you'll build up enough strength, and endurance to take on more intermediate movements.

Intermediate Training

When beginning intermediate training it is best to up the weight. If you want continuous results you must increase the difficulty to make sure that you continue gaining muscle.

The first on the list is _The Kettlebell Sit Up_. _The Kettlebell Sit Up_ is a very effective technique. It's a weighted abdominal exercise. People forget that abs are just like any muscle, using body weight alone won't be enough to make them pop out. If you want ab definition you have to increase the weight resistance. The Kettlebell is a great way of doing just that.

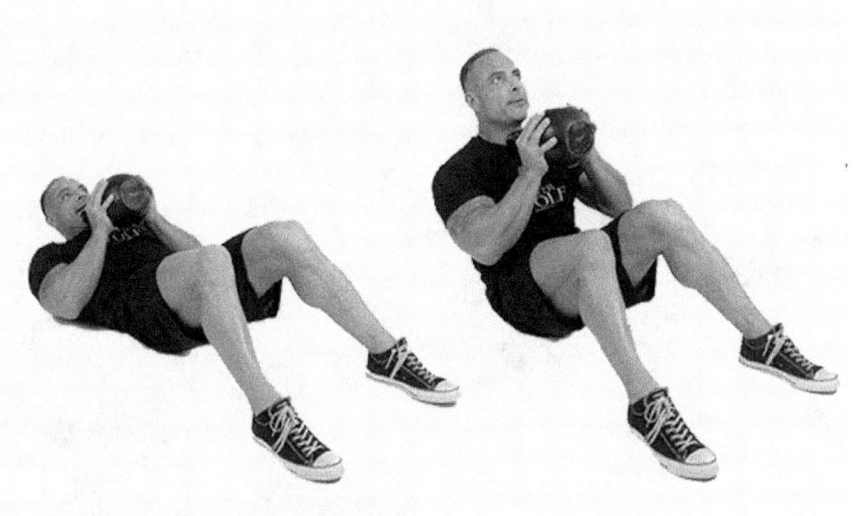

The next exercise is <u>*The Russian Twist*</u>. *The Russian Twist* is a classic kettlebell move. It's incredibly effective at working the obliques. If you don't want those pesky love handles *The Russian Twists* is the exercise for you. Take a look at the way she's holding the Kettlebell. As you can see she's keeping her back stable making sure not to lose control.

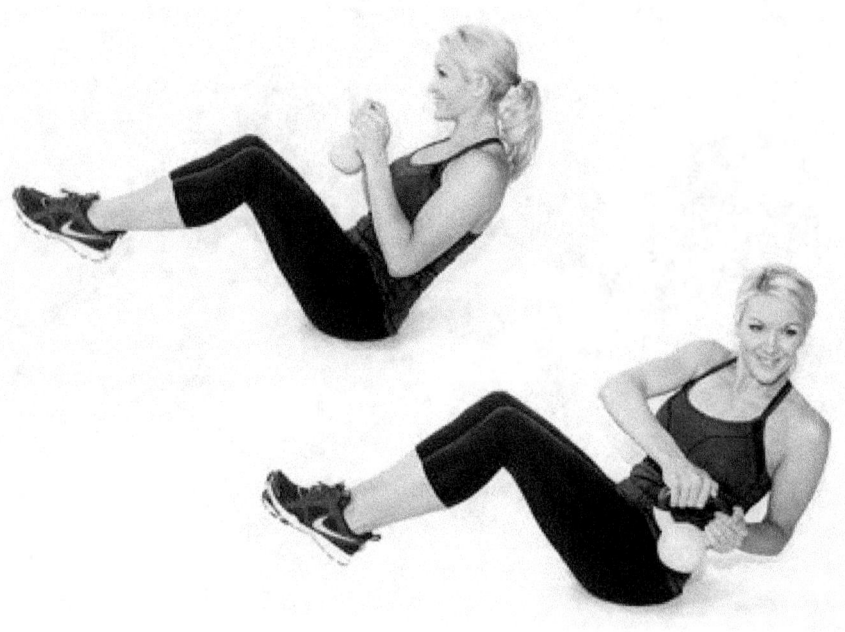

Next on the list is *The Figure Eight*. This is another exercise that's incredibly effective at working your abdominals. It also has the added benefit of working your hamstrings. Always keep your back straight so that you don't bend forward when you passed the Kettlebell between your legs.

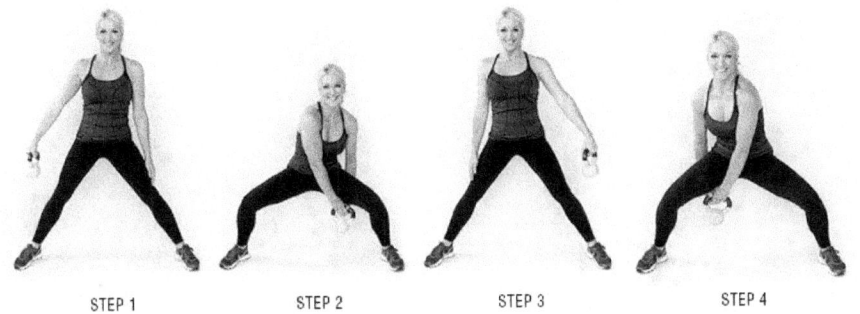

STEP 1   STEP 2   STEP 3   STEP 4

Next on the list is _The Two Handed Squat_. _The Two Handed Squat_ works the quadriceps, hamstrings, gluteus maximus, and erector spinae. It's a very simple move when you look at it, but with repetition your quads will start to burn.

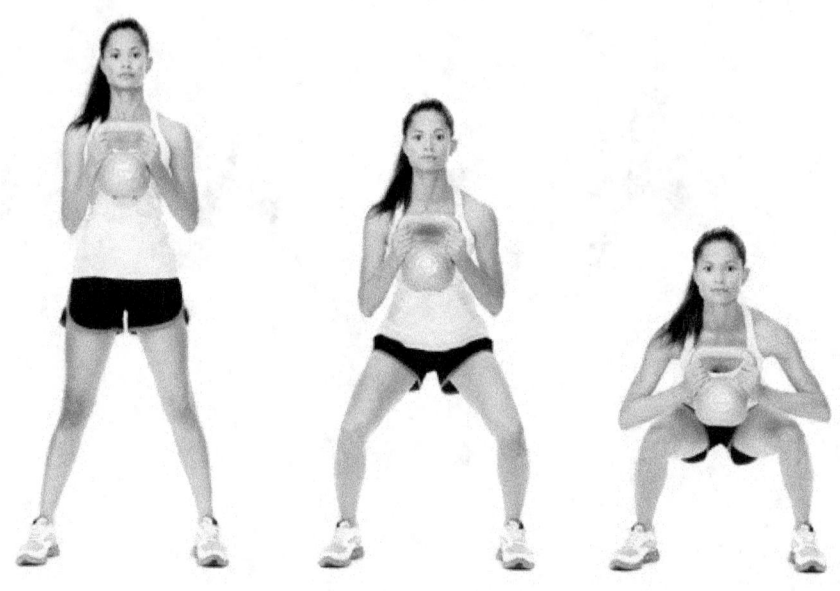

Next would be *The Squat & Press*. The *Squat & Press* is one of my favorite moves. It works the majority of the body. Glutes, hamstrings, quadriceps, core, back, and arms. It's a very simple compound movement, but it's incredibly effective.

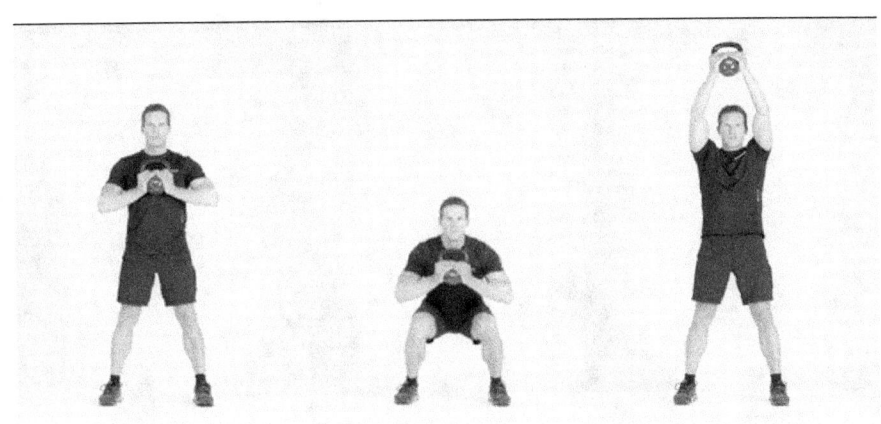

The next move is _The Clean_. The Clean works the majority of the body. You get to work your chest, your shoulders, your back, your biceps, triceps, your abs, legs, and glutes all in one move.

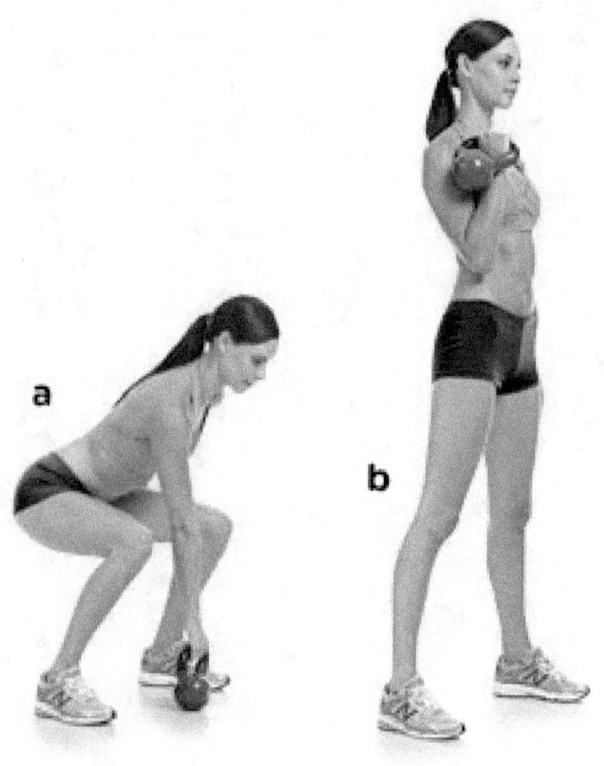

Next on the list is *The Snatch*. Now I know the name sounds a little funny, but the workout is actually incredibly effective. *The Snatch* works the hamstrings, quads, back, and shoulders. If you're looking to create stability in your body increasing your balance, and control the snatch is a good move to practice. If you look at the photo below you can see that the move is all about momentum.

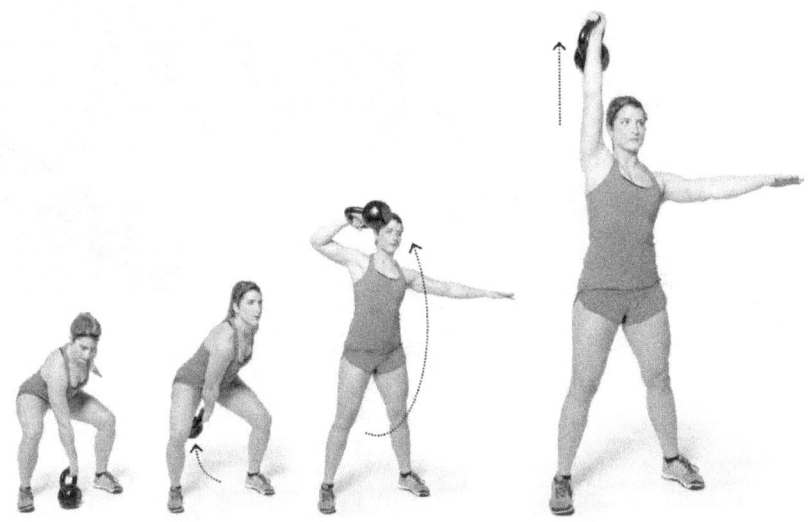

Next on the list is *The Lunge Row*. The Lunge Row is good for your rear shoulders, glutes, quads, side shoulders, triceps, biceps, hamstrings, lower back, and rhomboids. Just make sure to keep your back in a stable position, and pull your elbow as far back as you can. If you're looking to create extra strength in your back this is definitely one of the better kettlebell moves.

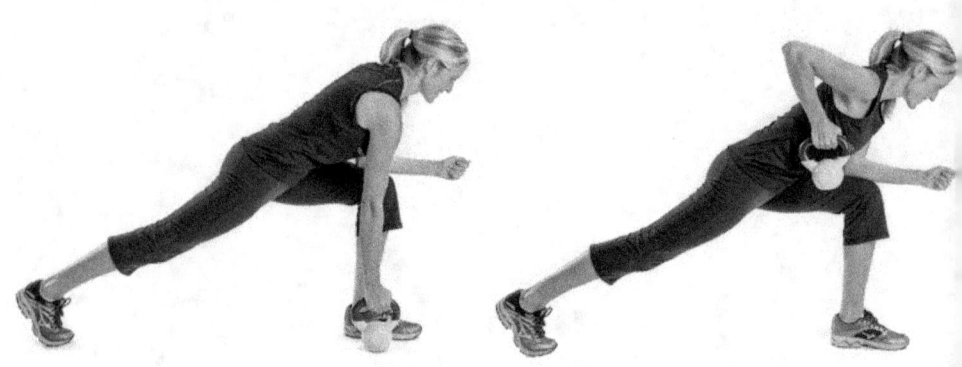

Next is *The Kettlebell One Arm Row*. *The One Arm Row* works the rear deltoids, trappe middle region, lats, and lower back. It's an incredibly effective yet incredibly simple movement. You just want to make sure you don't jerk the weight. Lift in a fluid, and controlled motion.

A   B

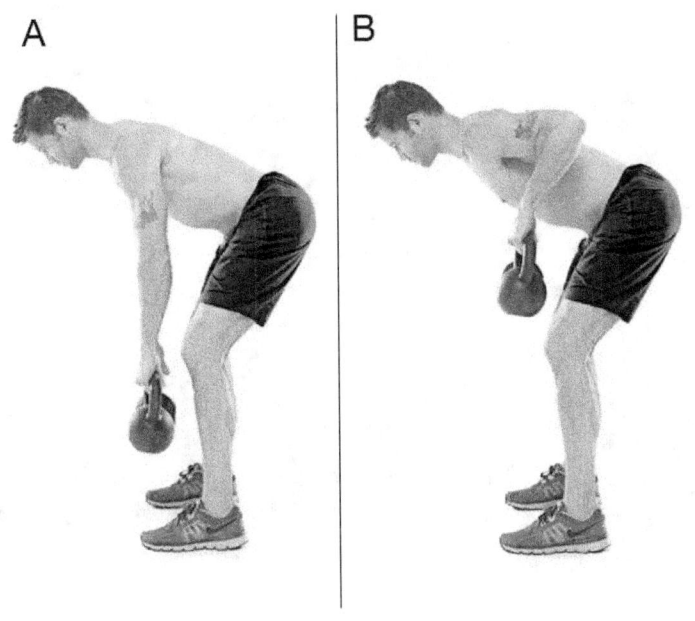

Next on the list is *The Lunge Press*. *The Lunge Press* is good for your thighs, core, and back. If you're looking for a strong intermediate workout to increase your leg strength this is the work out for you.

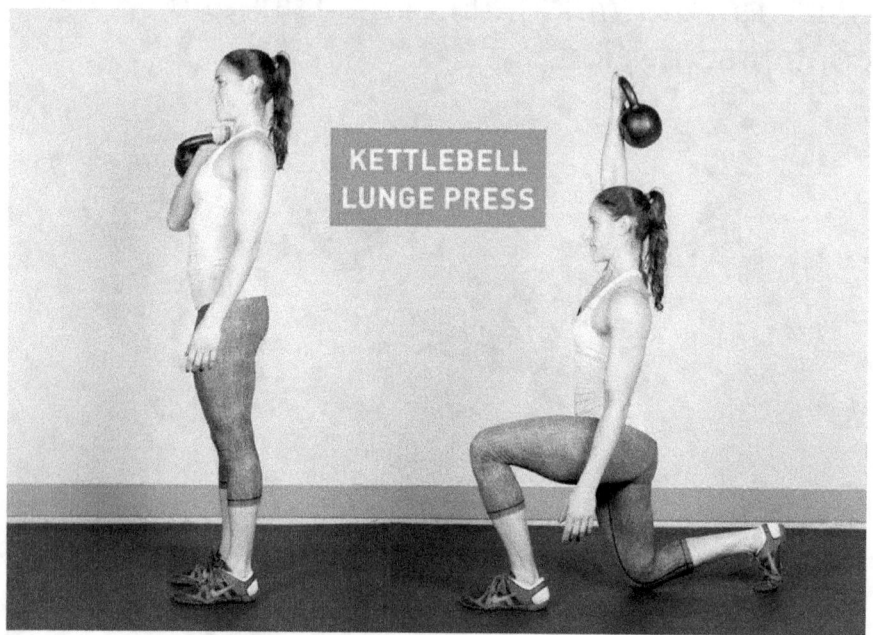

KETTLEBELL LUNGE PRESS

Next on our list is _The Bicep Curl_. As you probably already know _The Bicep Curl_ works the biceps. Try a one-arm bicep curl. You can grip the Kettlebell by the horns, and do a two arm bicep curl. The Bicep Curl is a good way to judge your strength. If you can do ten one arm bicep curls easily the weight is to light.

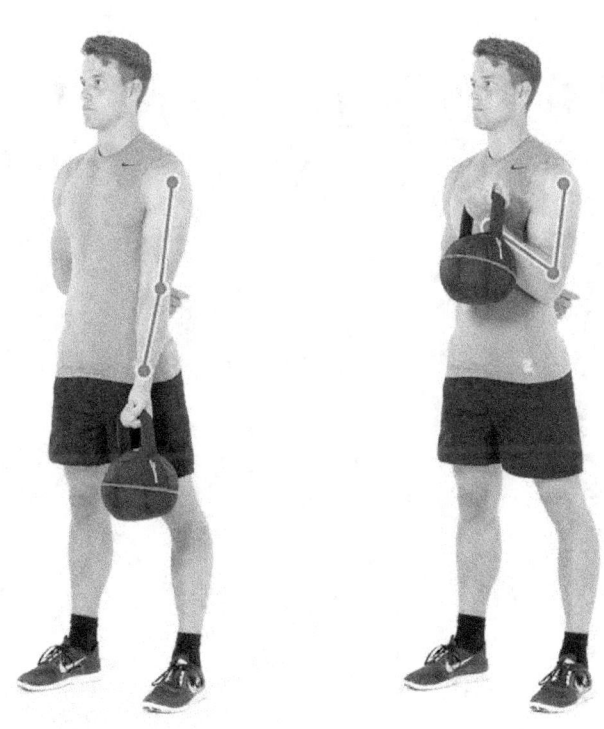

Next on our list is the rotating lunge. The rotating lunge works the obliques, ABS, quads, glutes, and hamstrings. The Move may look simple, but trust me balance is a key factor. When doing *The Rotating Lunge* you have to stabilize your core, back, and legs. It's a full-body stabilization workout making it great for stability, and balance enhancement. If you can do a set of these with out wobbling, my hat goes off to you.

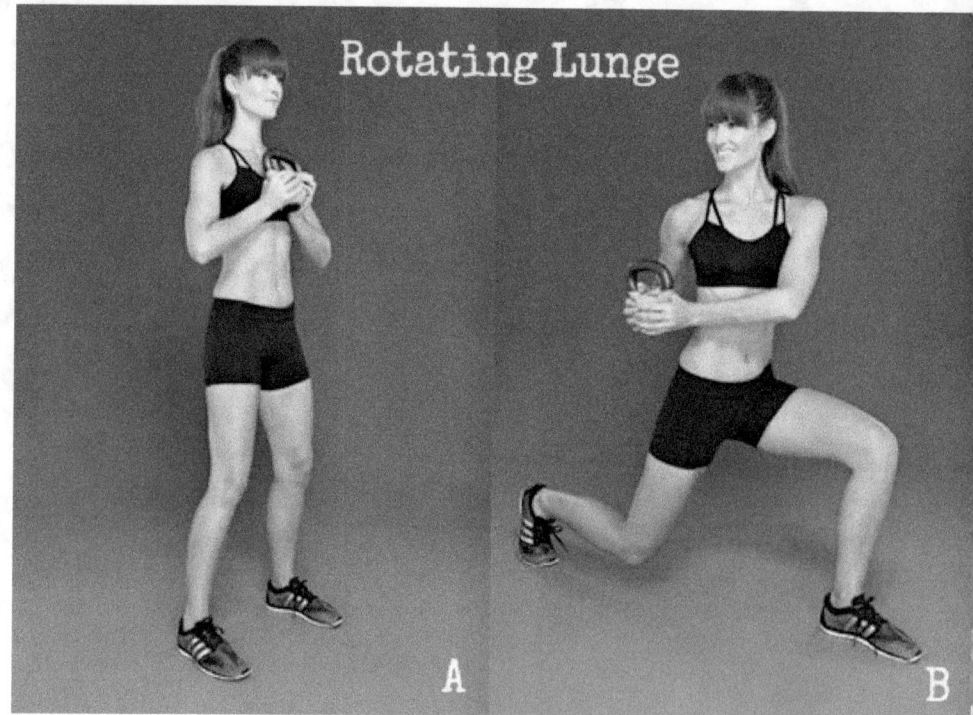

Rotating Lunge

A   B

Last but not least is _The Sumo Squat Lift._
Also called _The Sumo Squat High Pull_. _The
Sumo Squat Lift_ works the quads, glutes,
hamstrings, biceps, and upper back. It's one of
those incredible compound movements
targeting a large range of muscles.

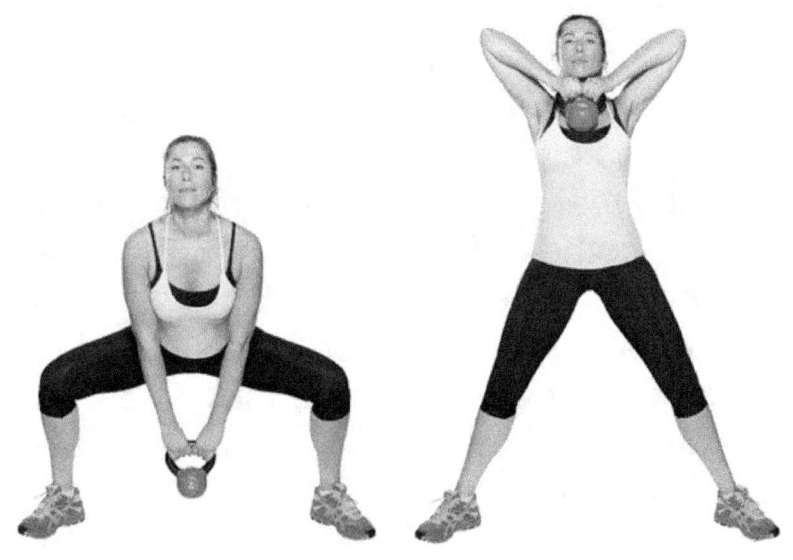

You can mix, and match these moves
together in any combination. Within a 36-
minute session you can do 2 minutes of each
one of these workouts. These intermediate
workouts will increase your core stability
allowing you a greater range of motion. They
will also increase your flexibility, and muscle
endurance. Do 36 minutes a day for 30 days.
In 30 days you should be ready to move on.

You're going to have more energy than you've ever had before.

Advance Training

Now that you're on an advanced level you may be thinking of upping the weight considerably. Be careful you want to make sure that you can handle the weight. If you get a kettlebell that's too heavy you might not be able to do some of the exercises in the advanced program. Therefore it might be best for you to only go up by 5 or 10 pounds at first. When you get the hang of the movements, and increase your strength you can increase the weight considerably.

The first move is _The Half Get Up_. _The Half Get Up_ is a very advanced move. It will require stability, and strength beyond any other move you've done so far. _The Half Get Up_ works the interior deltoid, erector spinae, external obliques, gluteus maximus, internal obliques, lateral deltoid, posterior deltoid, rectus abdominis, infraspinatus, and multifarious. It's truly a powerful move. The half get up requires an extremely large amount of abdominal strength. It's one of the most effective abdominal workouts, but it's also one of the most difficult.

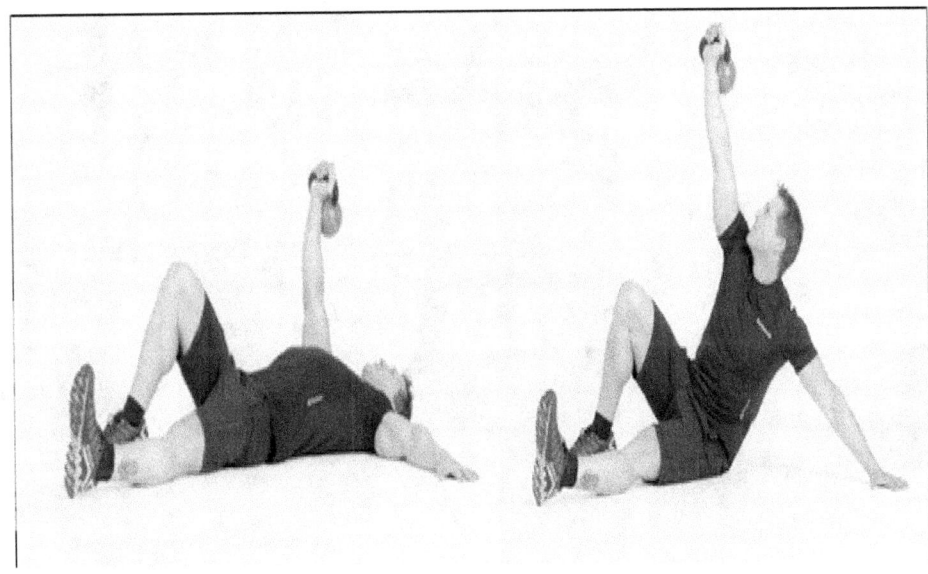

Next on the list is _The Turkish Get Up_.
The Half Get Up is just one piece of _The Turkish Get Up_. In my opinion _The Turkish Get Up_ is the most complex move. _The Turkish Get Up_ requires a greater range of motion, control, stability, and endurance than any other compound movement. It works every muscle that _The Half Get Up_ does including the quadriceps, traps, and hamstrings. Doing _The Turkish Get Up_ for 15 minutes is considered an advanced level workout.

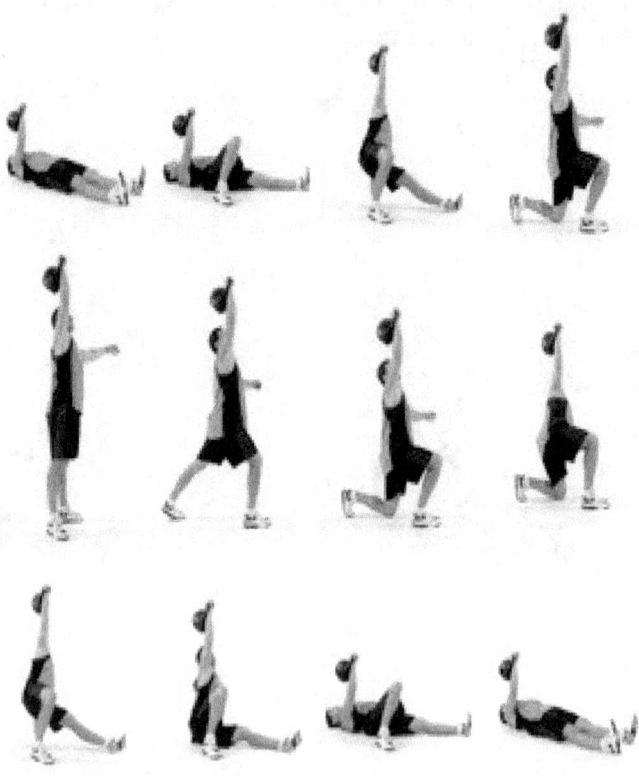

Next up is _The Single Leg Deadlift_. _The Single Leg Deadlift_ works the latissimus dorsai, abdominals, quadriceps, and hamstrings. It's important for balance. This move creates stability, and allows you to easily balance on one leg.

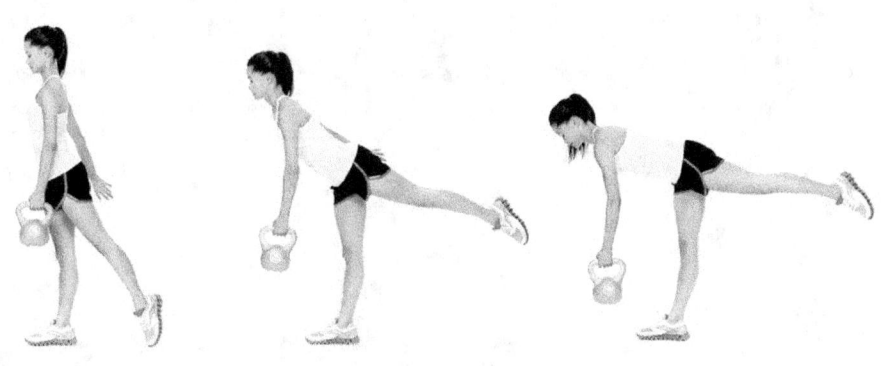

The next move is _The Overhead Jackknife_. _The Overhead Jackknife_ works the triceps, and the core. It's one of those core exercises that you can easily add into your routine. Just make sure to hold on to the weight you don't want it to drop on your face.

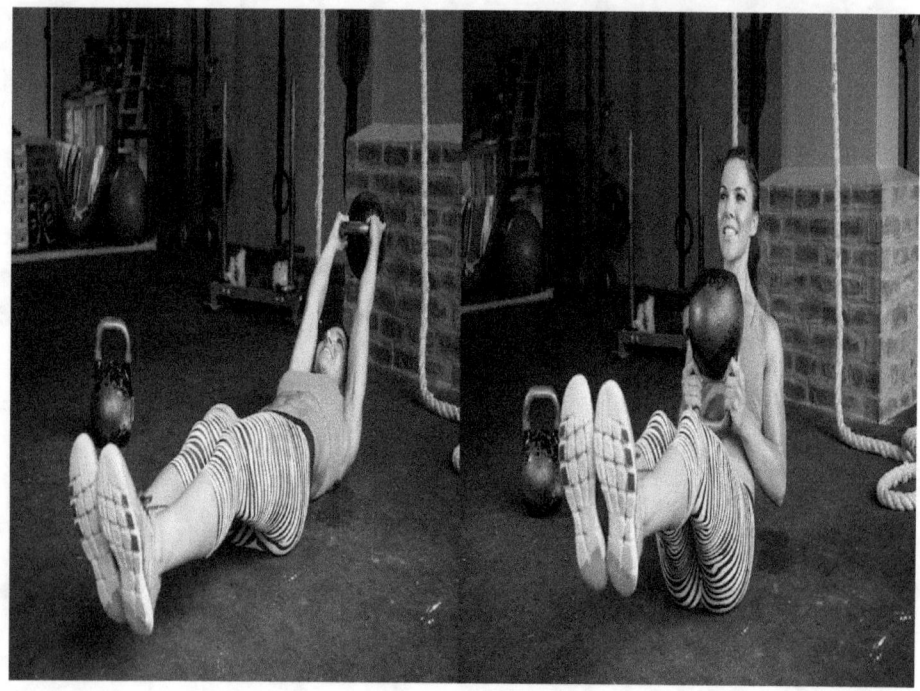

The next move is _The Chop_. _Chops_ work the latissimus dorsai, abdominals, quadriceps, and gluteus maximus. To be honest chops are one of the more fun moves to do. All my friends find them quite enjoyable. Although they can be quite fun if you don't keep your balance the move could be quite dangerous near fragile objects. Make sure to keep your back straight and control the weight.

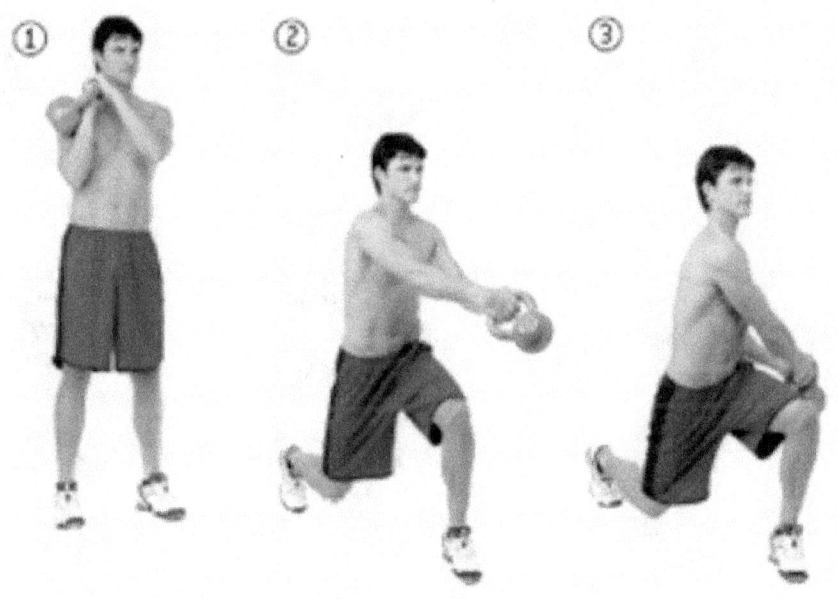

The next move is _The Clean & Press_.
The Clean & Press works the triceps, traps,
abdominals, calves, lower back, hamstrings,
and glutes. It's one of those advanced
compound movements that gives you an
almost full body workout. This move is
guaranteed to get you ready for the summer.

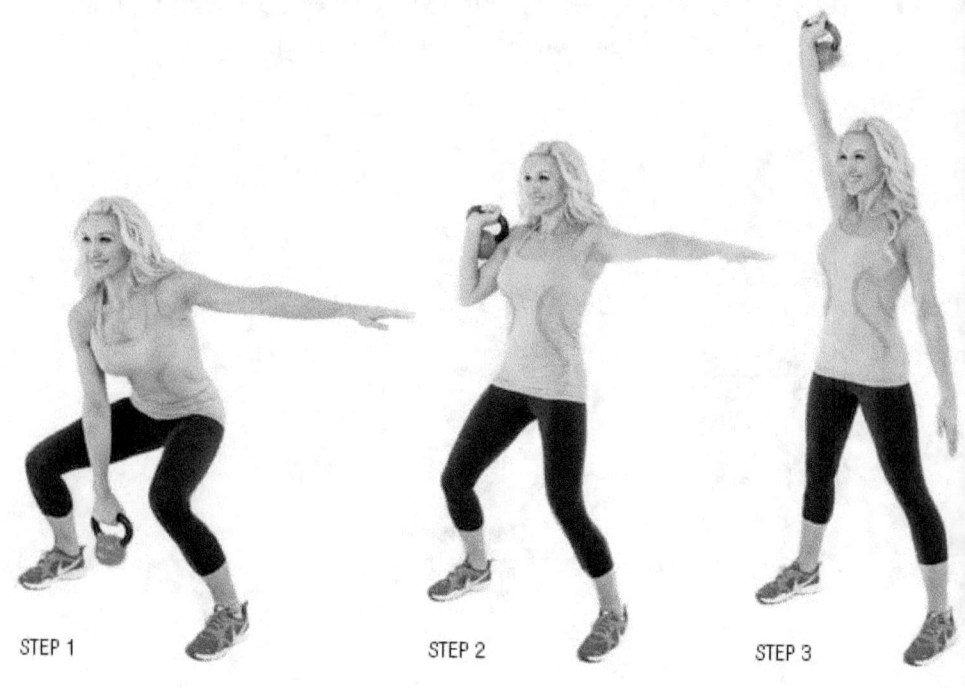

STEP 1   STEP 2   STEP 3

The next move is _The Two-Handed Deadlift_. This is a basic move unless you're lifting a heavy load. You have to make sure to stabilize your back otherwise you could be putting more stress on it than necessary. Remember to lift with your legs not your back or your arms. _The Two-Handed Deadlift_ works the calves, quads, hamstrings, gluteus maximus, arms, core, back, trapeze, and shoulders.

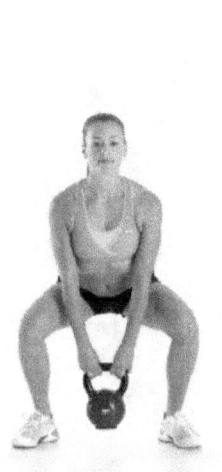
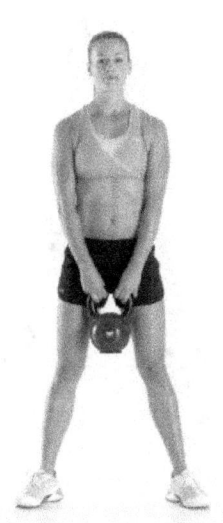

The next move is _The Windmill_. _The Windmill_ increases your flexibility significantly. It also works the shoulders, hamstrings, abdominals, and the gluteus maximus.

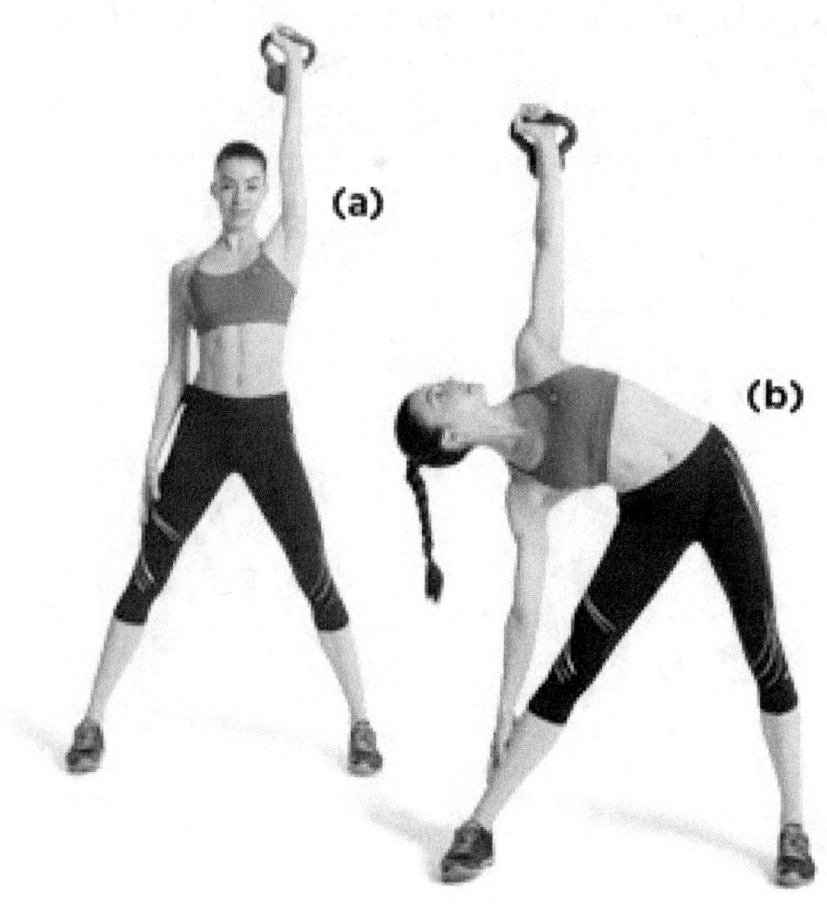

(a)

(b)

Next is *The Changing Hand Swing*. You're doing a one-arm kettlebell swing, but when you get to the top you grab the Kettlebell with your other hand. This move is very effective at strengthening your lower back, your shoulders, your gluteus maximus, your hips, hamstrings, and abdominals. *The Changing Hand Swing* is one of my go to moves. Usually if I'm in the middle of a routine, and I can't think of what to do next I just do the changing hand swing. It's truly a powerful compound workout.

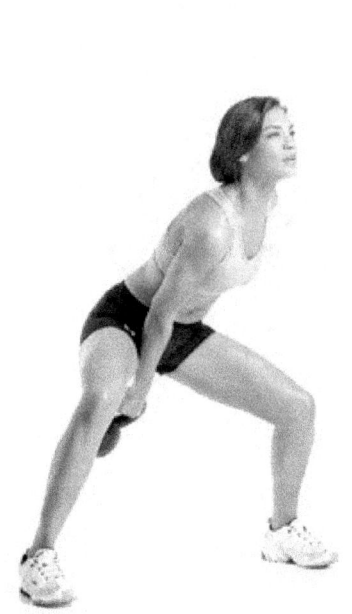
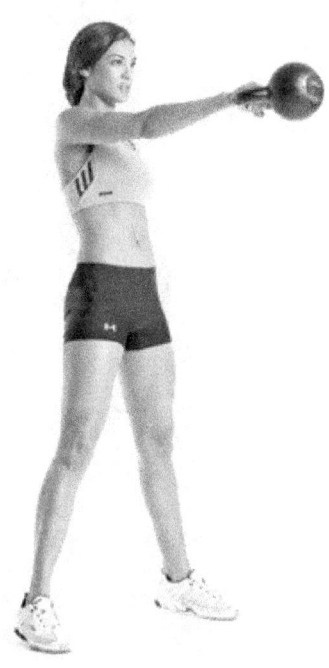

Next is *The Standing Twist*. This move is great for isolating those abdominals. You just need to make sure that you use a weight that you can control. You don't want to lean forward while you're doing the standing twist! It will cause unnecessary strain on your back.

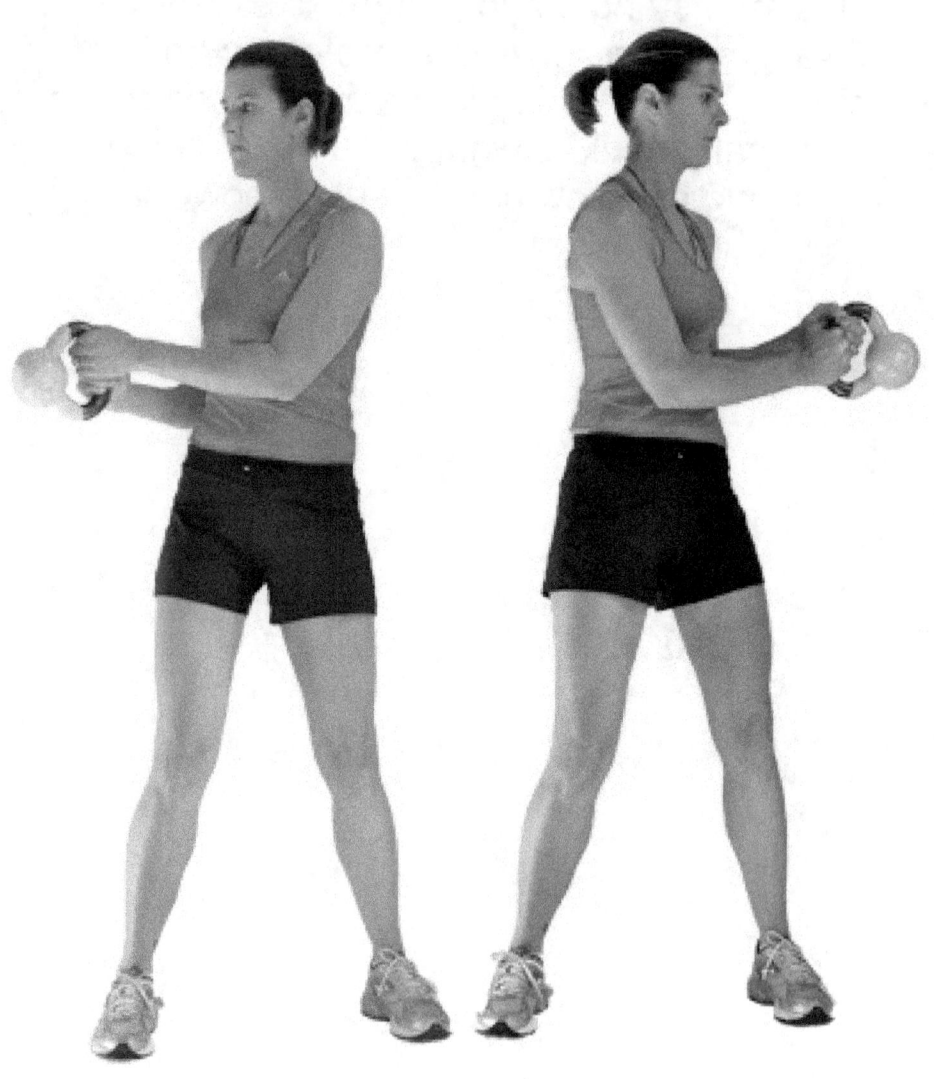

Next is *The One Arm Press*. *The One Arm Press* is looked at as a beginner move, but when doing it with heavy weight it becomes truly advanced. *The One Arm Press* works the shoulders, triceps, and core.

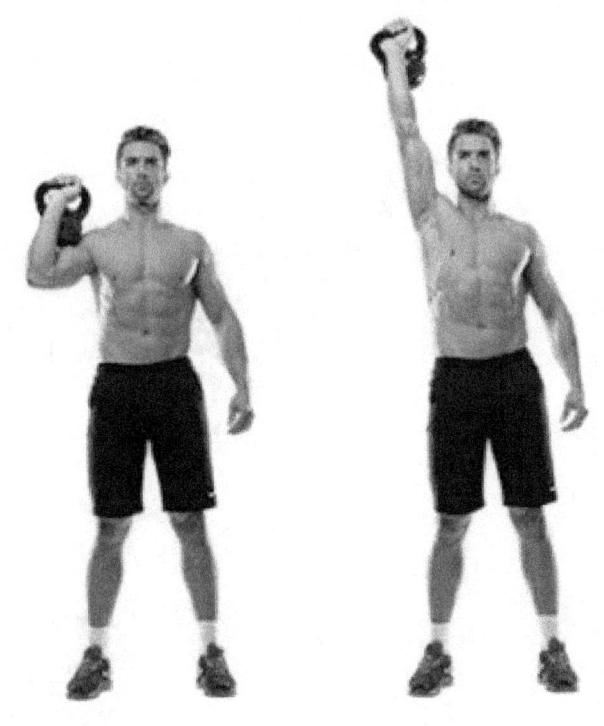

Next is _The Sit & Press_. _The Sit & Press_ works the core, and the arms. The move looks simple, but I assure you it is not. _The Sit & Press_ requires incredible core strength, and stability. You want to use a weight you can handle.

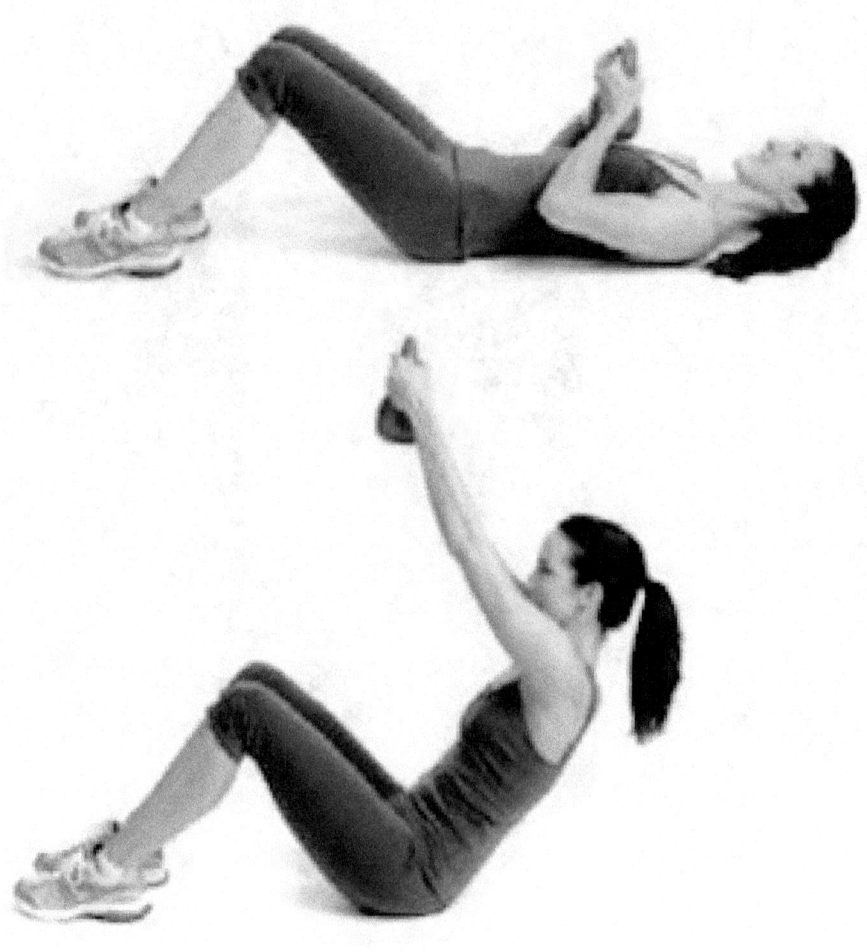

Next is *The Tricep Extension*. *The Tricep Extension* of course works the triceps. Depending on the weight it could be a very strenuous exercise. Make sure you hold on to the weight tightly you don't want to drop it on your head. Use your core to stabilize your body so that the weight doesn't move you backwards.

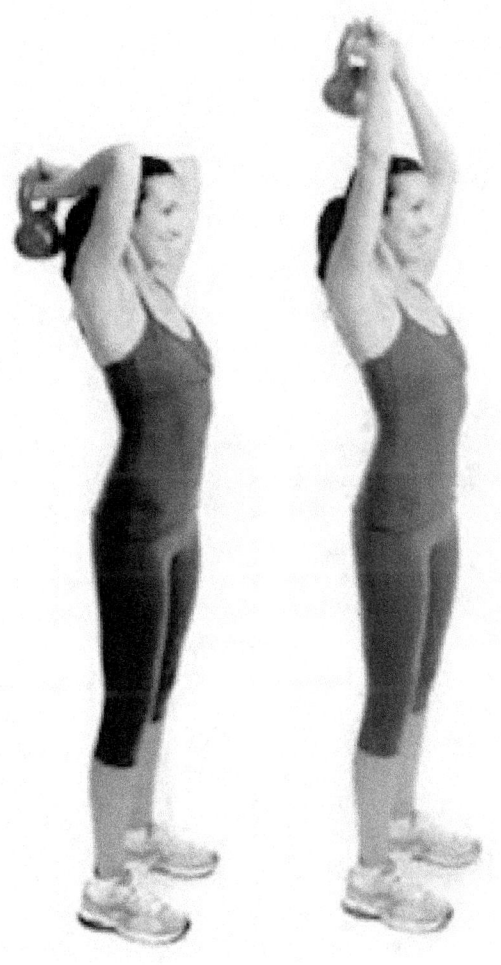

Next is _The Halo_. The Halo is one of my favorite kettlebell moves. It works the deltiods, the shoulders, the pecs, the chest, the triceps, and the abdominals. Looking at the move your probably thinking how could such a simple movement work so many muscles. Well this move isn't simple at all. Keeping control of a heavy kettlebell while twisting it around your head isn't a cakewalk. In my experience this really increases your core strength, and balance.

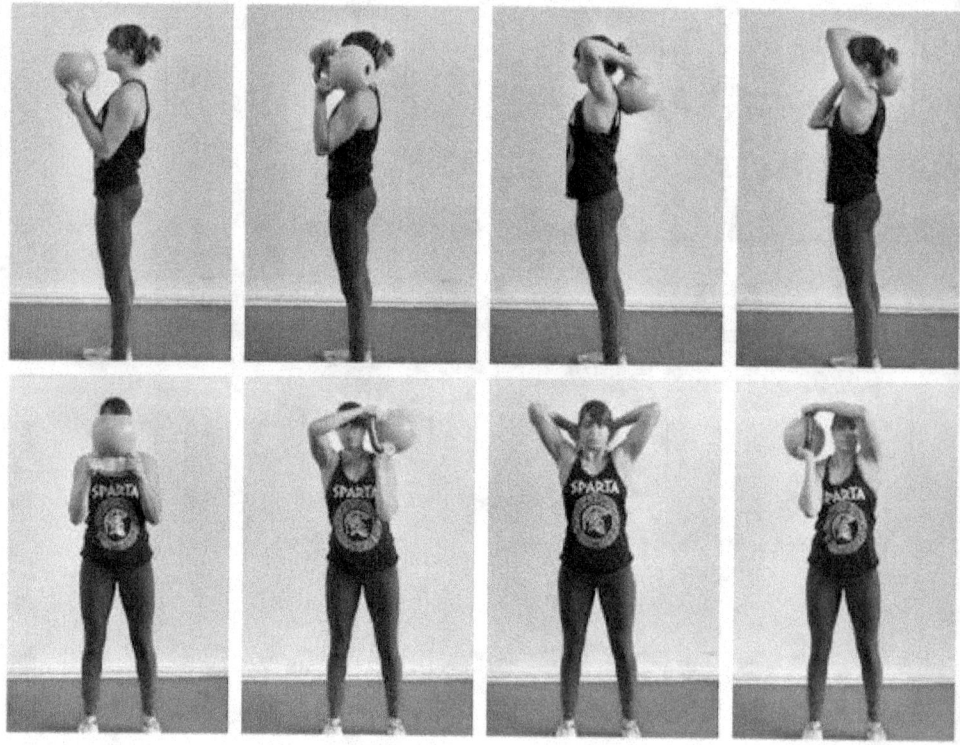

Next is _The Racked Squat_. Of course you would switch arms, and do this move on both sides. It works the quadriceps, the hamstrings, the gluteus maximus, and erector spinae.

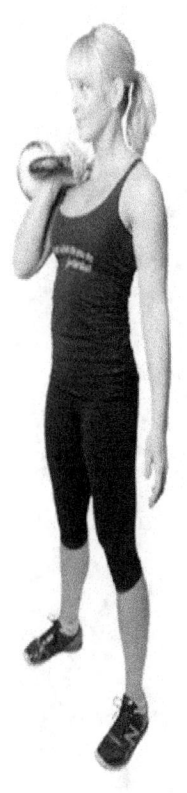
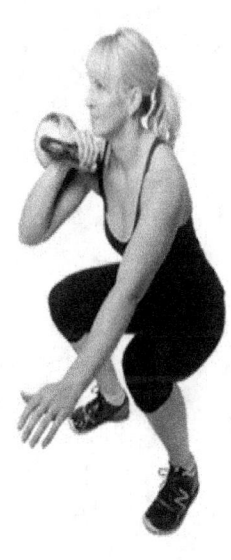

Next is *The Racked Reverse Lunge*. The *Rack Reverse Lunge* works the lower back, shoulders, abdominals, calves, gluteus maximus, and hamstrings. This is one of the best moves you can do to work pretty much every single muscle in your legs. It requires great balance, and stability so it's great for your core.

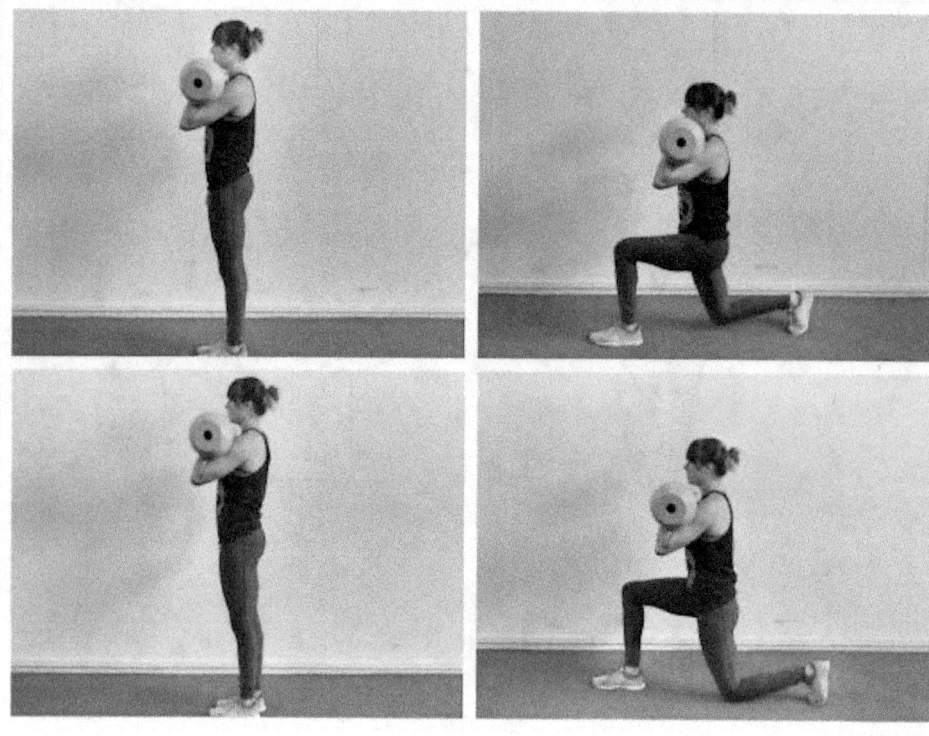

Next is *The Side Lunge & Clean*. *The Side Lunge & Clean* is a incredibly effective move. Any advance kettlebell user will tell you that this move works wonders for most every aspect of your body. *The Side Lunge & Clean* works the gluteus maximus, abductors, quads, hamstrings, soleus, tibias anterior, chest, shoulders, back, biceps, triceps, and abs. It's one of the most powerful compound movements in the Kettlebell world. 15 minutes of *The Side Lunge & Clean* is considered an advanced kettlebell workout.

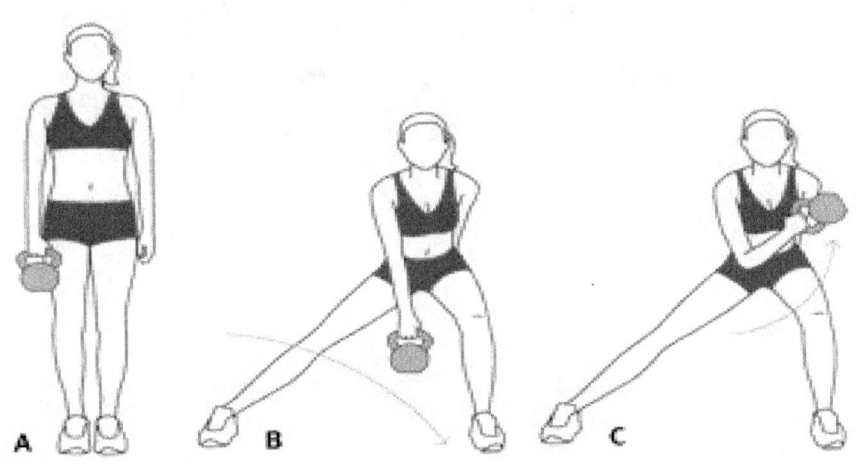

Next is *The One Leg Clean & Press*. This is a truly an advanced level move. When it comes to improving your balance, and stability no move is more effective. *The One Leg Clean & Press will push your balance to the limit. If you can do this without wobbling you have the balance of ah yoga master. Check it out here:* https://www.youtube.com/watch?v=vb-Aoow2zXc

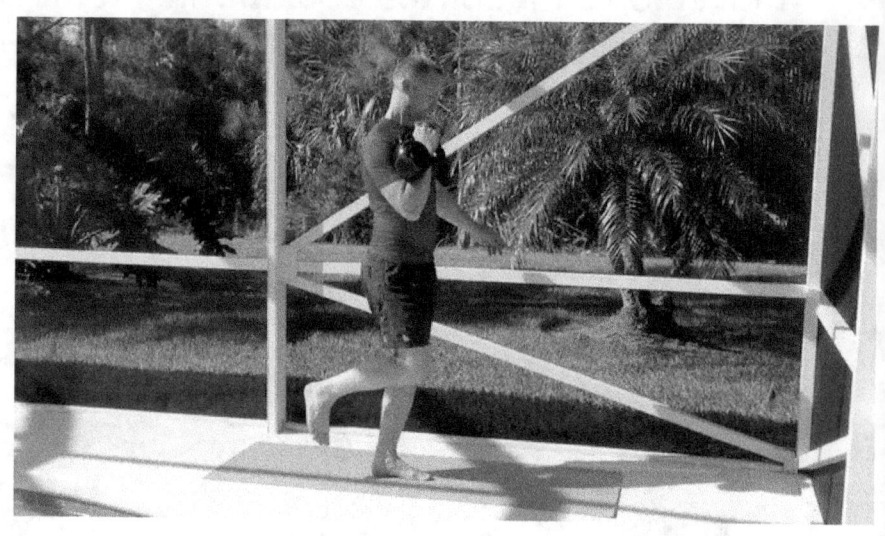

Next is *The Clean Squat Press*. *The Clean Squat Press* works the shoulders, traps, triceps middle lower back, abdominals, gluten, quadriceps, hamstrings, and calves. It's an interesting compound movement that works pretty much every major muscle group in the body.

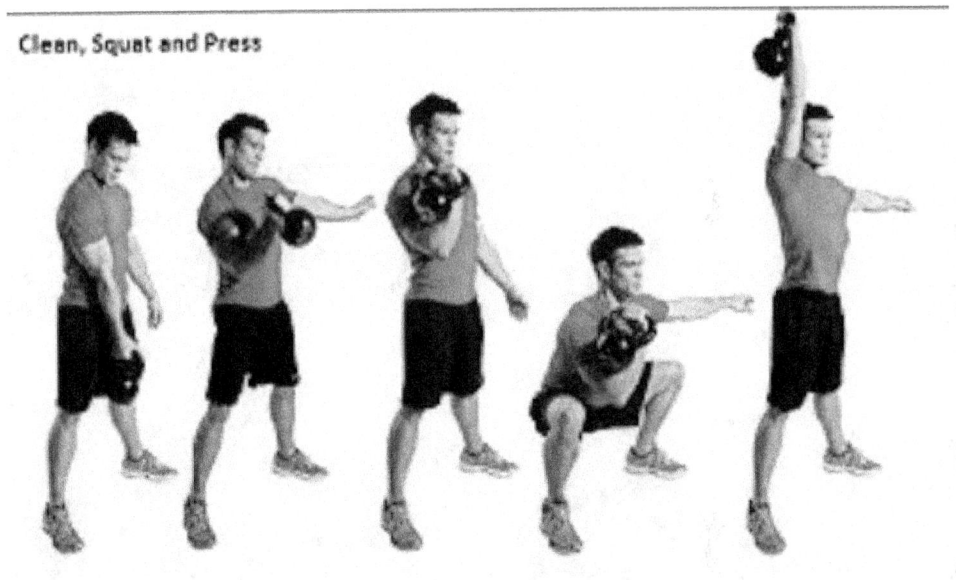

Clean, Squat and Press

Next is *The Lateral Swing*. *The Lateral Swing* is a complex movement that requires extreme control. If you think you're going to let go of the Kettlebell for one second than you need to stop. *The Lateral Swing* will cut body fat like a steak knife. If you combine *The Kettlebell Swing* with *The Changing Hand Swing,* and *The Lateral Swing* you got yourself a 30-minute workout that will have you ready for summer!

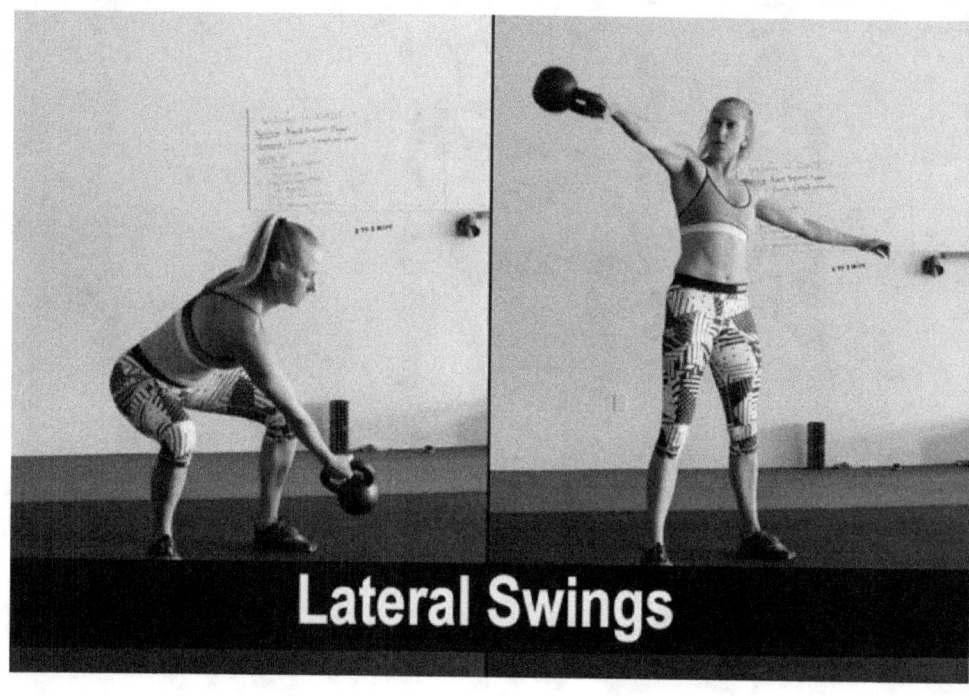

Lateral Swings

Last but not least is <u>*The Pistol Squat*</u>. I put *The Pistol Squat* last because to me it is the most difficult move. *The Pistol Squat* works the hips, hamstrings, quadriceps, gluteus maximus, and calves. It's the most effective workout to do when trying to strengthen individual legs. If you can't do *The Pistol Squat* without the Kettlebell don't try it with the Kettlebell.

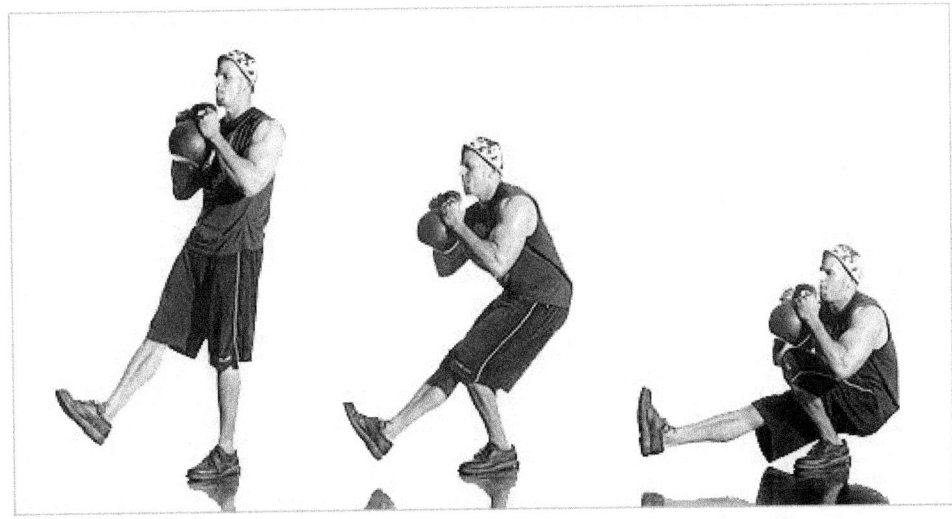

These advanced level workouts will have you ready for anything. The Kettlebell works out the entire body from head to toe building plenty of muscle endurance. You'll notice you have plenty of energy, stamina, and focus throughout the day. The Kettlebell is a time-tested tool. It's more ancient than any workout machine in any gym. To be exact the kettlebell is from the 1700s. An hour of any Kettlebell workout burns 1200 calories. There are 3500 calories in a pound so three hours of kettlebell burns a pound! How about that!

Motivation

All it takes is motivation. With motivation we all move forward. With motivation we overcome our weaknesses, and take control of our destinies. If there's anything in your life that has held you back allow the thought of you overcoming, and rising above it to motivate you. Allow the thought of better health to become a reality. With better health we all look at life differently. The more exercise that we offer our body the better our mind works. If we know what's negative in our life than we know what the sickness is. There are millions of people in this world that don't know what their problem is. They have no way of identifying the true issues that plagues their body. If you can look in the mirror, and stare your problem right in the face than you have something that they don't, and that's hope. You can hope for a better tomorrow because you can identify the problem. If you can identify the problem than you can find a solution. If your problem is lack of energy, strength, and coordination _The Kettlebell Cleanse_ is the solution. If your problem is obesity _The Kettlebell Cleanse_ is the solution. In this world very few people get to see the best version of themselves. Become the best version of you mentally, and physically, and watch the world around you change. When I became the best version of myself physically, and mentally, I became a different person. It's not all about the physical progression that you make. It's about the feeling the bell gives you. You will start to feel great in so many different ways. The way the bell made me feel was my guiding light. Every day I woke up happy, healthier, and cheerful. For once it felt like I did something to change my circumstances. At times I felt as if the hand dealt to me was permanent, and that there was nothing that I could do. After trying so many different avenues I begin to understand that weight loss is much more complex. Infomercials made it seem easy. Get this product, and you'll be ready for summer in a month. The truth is nothing like that exists. It's an unfortunate realization.

Body fat percentage is everything. Being a 200-pound man could mean anything depending on your body fat percentage. If your 6 foot 2 200 pounds 50% body fat that's not good! If your 6 foot 2 200 pounds 12% body fat that's amazing. The deciding factor is your body fat percentage. How much of your body is muscle, and how much of your body is fat. The more you tip the scale towards muscle the easier it is for you to lose fat, and keep it off. A lot of people talk about turning fat into muscle, but there is no such thing. If you're trying to gain muscle you eat more calories than your body requires while lifting weights. If you're trying to lose fat you eat less calories than your body requires while lifting weights. The problem is people use cardio equipment to try to lose weight. The issue with this is this type of exercise burns muscle, and fat indiscriminately. When using the treadmill you're not building muscle, but you are using energy. Your body is looking for a fuel source so that you can continue to run. It will get it from muscle, or fat. Compare that to a weighted cardio exercise. In this case you're actually using your muscles. So instead of you burning muscle, and fat you'll be preserving muscle, and burning fat. You want to lose weight without losing muscle.

Let's say you are a female, and your 5 foot 6 200 pounds 40% body fat. You lose 40 pounds doing cardio. Now you're 5 foot 6 160 pounds 50% body fat. That's still going to look bad. Body fat percentage is what's important not how much you weigh. If you lose that same 40 pounds with the Kettlebell your body fat percentage is going to go down. If you're 160 pounds, and you're 40% body fat 64 pounds of you is pure fat the rest is lean muscle. Now let's pretend that you lost this weight using the Kettlebell. You go from 200 to 160, but you've lost nothing, but pure body fat, and just a little muscle. This means your 160 pounds, and 25% body fat. That's going to look wonderful. You want to hold on to your muscle, and get rid of your fat. That's the key to genuine weight loss. You can make all of this happen if you stay motivated, and follow the program. Mix and match these exercises 5 days a week for 30 minutes to an hour. I guarantee you'll see, and feel the difference. You just have to stay motivated.

Vitamin Intake

Let me start this off by saying that by no means am I telling you to buy any of these vitamins. I'm just telling you the vitamins that I used during _The Kettlebell Cleanse_. I have no idea if they had an effect on my results, but I feel like they're worth mentioning. My vitamin intake during _The Kettlebell Cleanse_ was well rounded. I tried to make sure I covered every single function of my body. Let's start things off with the first vitamin I took.

Ubiquinol is said to be very good for your cardiovascular health, and the last thing I wanted going out on me was my heart because I had high blood pressure. Ubiquinol was a supplement I took to make sure I had a little extra energy. Its supposed to be an incredibly powerful antioxidant it's also supposed to promote energy production as well, and I needed all the energy that I could get. They say it's good for brain health, and protecting the cells from free radicals. To be honest I still use ubiquinol it's much better than

Co q-10 because it's easily absorb into the body.

The second thing I kind of supplemented with was _Apple Cider Vinegar With Mother_. I mixed my apple cider vinegar with a teaspoon of lemon juice, eight ounces of water, and made sure to take this every single day at least 2 times a day. I have no idea what kind of effect it may have had on my progression. I just know that it's still apart of my routine to this day. Apple cider vinegar is supposed to promote weight loss. I have no idea if it contributed to my weight loss, but I feel like it's worth mentioning.

The third supplement that I used was _Black Seed Oil_. Black seed oil is supposed to be the God of all supplements. It's supposed to promote health across the board. They say that it's a huge anti-inflammatory. Since pretty much every health problem is caused by inflammation black seed oil is probably the number one vitamin you can use. They say black seed oil is wonderful for cancer prevention and treatment. They also say it's crucial to liver health. They say that it prevents diabetes. They also say it's great for weight loss which was one of the main reasons why I started using it. They say that it's great for your hair, nails, and skin. They also say that it's wonderful for fighting off infections, and that it's effective against certain strains of superbugs that most antibiotics are not working on anymore. Black seed oil has been studied over, and over again. It's probably one of the most studied supplements on the market so there's some solid science to back up what it does. Still I have no idea if it had a major effect on my workout or not nor do I have any idea if it helped my weight loss.

Another supplement I used was _Grapeseed, Green Tea, & Pine Bark Complex_. The combination of these creates a super antioxidant. The main reason why I was taking it was for energy. The combination of these three things promotes a natural boost in energy. It's not like a caffeine pill or anything like that it's something that works overtime. This is one of those supplements that I don't like running out of I try to make sure that I keep it in stock as much as I possibly can.

I used *Probiotics* because they support your immune system. They're supposed to introduce positive bacteria back into your stomach. This is supposed to help your digestive system, and promote weight loss. I can say that I got sick a lot less often once I start taking the probiotics. Still I started sprinting around the same time so I can't really say which one was super effective.

L-Carnitine was one of the first supplements that I started using. It aids in transforming fat into energy. This is the most important process in weight loss, and energy production. Also it's supposed to aid in muscle building as well. It's supposed to be one of the main elements of muscle building. A lot of bodybuilders use L-Carnitine, and some even say it helps with your overall brain health. Now I don't know if it did any of these things for me I just know during *The Kettlebell Cleanse* I took it everyday.

Omega-3 Fish Oil is something that I've been taking since I was a kid. It's supposed to support cardiovascular health, and cognitive function. It supports your immune system, your bone health, and your joint health as well. It's also said to support a healthy mood. I don't know if it does any of these things I just know that my mom has been giving me omega-3 fish oil since I was a kid. It's supposed to be one of the most important vitamins on the planet for preserving your body, and promoting overall health.

Vitamin D3 is a supplement I started taking when I realize that I probably wasn't getting enough of it. Vitamin D comes from sun exposure, and since I don't really go outside too often I knew that I probably was vitamin D3 deficient. Vitamin D3 is supposed to support bone destiny, the immune system, and boost absorption of calcium. It's supposed to support neuromuscular function whatever that means. All I know is Vitamin D3 is very important to the body, and if you're not getting enough sunlight than most likely you're not getting enough vitamin D3. Still I have no idea if it had any effect on my performance whatsoever.

Biotin is something that I also supplemented with. It's supposed to be good for your hair, nails, and skin. It's also supposed to support some other viable functions in the body. I guess biotin is one of the key ingredients that your hair needs to grow. That's one of the main reasons why I was supplementing with it. I will say when I started to use it I did notice a difference in my hair quality, nail quality, and the appearance of my skin. It took about three to four months though. Still I'm not sure if that was the sprinting or the biotin or a combination of both.

Sea kelp was something else that I used. It's supposed to be a source of iodine. Iodine is important for thyroid function. The thyroid regulates a huge amount of functions in your body including your hormonal balance. Your hormonal balance has a huge effect on your energy levels, your mood, and also your weight. If your thyroid isn't functioning properly than most likely you're going to have weight issues. They say this is why the Japanese are so skinny because their diet is rich in iodine. It's because they eat so much seaweed. Still I have no idea if it had any effect on my weight loss.

Garcinia Cambogia is supposed to stop your body from creating new fat. It was featured on Dr. Oz a while ago, and it's supposed to be proven to actually stop your body from creating new fat. Now I'm not sure if it stopped my body from creating new fat all I know is that it was a part of my everyday regimen.

Of course I took a _Multi Vitamin_ because that just makes common sense. Everybody probably takes a multi-vitamin I've been taking one since I was a kid. It's always been apart of my regimen.

African Mango was also something that I included in my supplement regimen. It's supposed to help promote weight loss but there isn't much research behind it to say that it does anything of any kind of significance. Still a lot of people swear by it so I added it to my supplement pile.

I also took _L-Theanine_, and if you're a coffee drinker like me L-Theanine is absolutely essential. It gets rid of that jittery affect that coffee gives you, and makes it a smooth high. It also has some other benefits that might be worth mentioning. Apparently in 1964 Japan approved L-Theanine for unlimited use in all foods. L-Theanine has been linked to relieving stress. It's the key ingredient in green tea, which has been linked to relieving stress.

I'm not endorsing any of these vitamins in anyway. I'm just informing you of the supplements I used during *The Kettlebell Cleanse*. These supplements may have enhanced my results, and it wouldn't be fair if I didn't mention them. If you choose to take them my best advice is to have a conversation with your doctor. If you want to know the exact supplements that I used than check out my website http://workoutkingrule.blogspot.com/.

Mind Your Diet

If you don't pay attention to what you eat you're not going to be able to accomplish anything. In this situation I'm speaking about eating for energy not eating for weight loss. Remember *The Kettlebell Cleanse* takes a lot of energy. If you're not eating for energy than you're not going to be able to last for very long. Your body is going to need power so therefore you have to eat the foods that give you the most power. I'm going to give you a detailed example of the type of foods I ate during *The Kettlebell Cleanse*. You can either mimic this, or find similar foods that might give you the drive you need.

First thing in the morning I made sure to blend a shake. I blended kale, oranges, apples, bananas, blueberries, cranberries, strawberries, and I used apple juice instead of water. I did research on each one of these fruits, and vegetables to make sure that they would give me the optimum performance that I was seeking.

Kale is the healthiest vegetable you can eat. I made sure to put more kale in my shake than anything else. Every single fruit that I mention I used a whole one. I used a whole orange, a whole apple, and ah whole banana. I used about maybe eight cranberries, eight blueberries, and about four strawberries. To be honest after I took the shake in the morning I always would feel wonderful. It was probably the best part of my diet, and a great way to kick off my day. I also had oatmeal because I wanted to make sure that I was getting an extreme amount of fiber.

The combination of these fruits and vegetables gave me an extreme amount of energy. It's probably the one thing that I can attest to my newfound power. It actually boosts my energy level. I don't know if any of my vitamins did anything to actually boost my energy level, but I'm sure my shake did the job. To be honest over time it became even more effective. Most people don't understand that eating healthy is something that takes time to affect your body. Sometimes you'll be able to feel it right away, but a lot of people quit because they don't feel any difference within a few days, or a week. I noticed after a month of taking the shake my overall mood in general changed. Remember I told you I was a very tired, cranky, and moody individual. I was so overweight my body had absolutely no energy whatsoever. When your body has no energy it pretty much ruins everything. You don't want to do anything. I can say that this shake had a profound effect on that mindset, and was a key ingredient in making _The Kettlebell Cleanse_ much more effective. I made sure that I didn't add any sugar to the mix. I also made sure to put cinnamon in my oatmeal. The cinnamon had a profound effect on my health as well. Remember cinnamon is nothing but pure fiber, and fiber is incredibly important to the digestive system. As long as you're going to the bathroom often you're losing weight. You want to make sure you're getting as much fiber as you possibly can. That's why I added apples to the mix because apples are rich in fiber. It's also why I added blueberries to the mix because they're rich in fiber as well. I wanted to make sure that I upped my fiber intake by as much as I possibly could. I also wanted to make sure I was getting a ton of vitamin C.

Vitamin C is the reason why I made sure to add a whole orange. I added bananas to the mix because I wanted to make sure that I was getting a lot of potassium. Bananas are good for Vitamin B6. Vitamin B6 is something that you'll see in almost every natural energy supplement.

Cranberries were just another source of fiber. They have even more fiber than blueberries. They're also packed full of antioxidants. The strawberries were mostly for flavor at first until I started doing more research, and I realize that strawberries were amazing. They can help prevent heart disease, stroke, cancer, high blood pressure, constipation, allergies, asthma diabetes, and depression. Strawberries are ah incredibly effective antioxidant.

Oatmeal is packed full of iron it's probably one of the most iron rich foods out there. It also has an extremely large amount of vitamin B6, magnesium, and vitamin A not to mention 6 grams of protein. Speaking of protein maybe I should discuss what I had for lunch.

Everyday for lunch I would have grilled chicken, beans, and a protein shake. My lunch was all about protein intake. For lunch I wanted to make sure I was getting as much protein in my body as possible. That's why I made sure I had grilled chicken because chicken has an extremely large amount of protein. Chicken is one of the most protein rich meats on the planet, and it's healthier for you than beef or pork. Not to mention it's a lot easier to cook especially if you know how to bake. It's even easier if you have a griller like one of those commercial grillers that drain out all the grease. Everyday when I woke up in the morning I would turn on my rice cooker, and add one cup or two cups of black beans. I chose black beans because they're low in calories. One cup is only 624 calories, and because they are extremely high in dietary fiber, you get 29 grams in one cup. Also because they're high in protein you get 39 grams of protein in one cup. They have an extremely large amount of iron, and ah extremely large amount of magnesium, and calcium so it was an obvious choice. Black beans are ah incredibly healthy super food with 2760 mg of potassium.

The body is supposed to consume at least 30 to 38 grams of fiber every day if you're a man. If you're a woman it's about 25 grams of fiber everyday. So basically one cup of black beans would almost be enough fiber for the day for a man and more than enough for a woman. If you read up on black beans you'll understand just how nutritious they really are. It's one of the most underestimated super foods on the planet. The only substitute that I would ever use for black beans if I didn't have them is quinoa. Quinoa is probably the greatest food on the planet, and the only food that has pretty much all the amino acids that you need. I also made sure that I had a whey protein isolate shake everyday.

For dinner I ate pretty much anything I wanted. I just made sure that I didn't eat any fast food. I completely cut out fast food in general. For dinner I would have a meal with black beans on the side. I would have ground turkey meat, chicken, or fish. I wouldn't have any beef or pork. So I would have some turkey tacos with black beans, and cheese, or I would have some turkey nachos with black beans, and cheese. Sometimes I would eat some salmon, beans, and rice. As long as I added the black beans to the meal I would create any combination I wanted. Eating beans with your meal helps the digestive process. It increases the nutritional value of the meal. I didn't really eat any dessert, but I've never been one to eat dessert anyway so it wasn't a big change for me.

My diet wasn't too extreme it wasn't anything that was impractical. All my food was good it wasn't like I had to eat nasty stuff that I didn't like. When you have to eat a bunch of nasty stuff that you don't like eventually you're going to give up on it. I loved the food I was eating! My shake was delicious, and my oatmeal was always good especially with cinnamon. I never put sugar in my oatmeal I just added cinnamon to it. If I wanted it to taste good I would add some honey. I made sure that I got my honey from the whole food store. Black beans are my favorite especially once you season them with some Lawry's, and some pepper. The grilled chicken was always good because I mean grilled chicken is awesome. Sometimes I would grill chicken and have a chicken black bean salad. It tasted great! My diet gave me energy, power, and change my mood all together. It's the main reason why I was able to go on. If I never changed my diet I would have never saw any positive effects from *The Kettlebell Cleanse* in the first place because I wouldn't be able to do it. My intention was never to change my diet for weight loss, but to promote energy production. I simply wanted to feel better, and run longer, and this diet accomplished that for me. I didn't find it difficult. If you can find food that has similar nutritious value that you actually find delicious by all means go about it in your own way. I'm just telling you exactly what I did. I don't want to leave any details out because that might be the one detail that contributed to my progression. If you choose to follow my diet to the letter it is more likely that you will see the same results that I did. Maybe you might find some loopholes that I didn't find. You might be able to improve upon the diet. If so please don't hoard information comment, and add your perspective. Tell the people of the dietary changes you implement that worked in combination with *The Kettlebell Cleanse.* Maybe tells us some of the vitamins that you used in combination with *The Kettlebell Cleanse*. Share other forms of kettlebell training you've tried in combination with *The Kettlebell Cleanse* that worked for you.

Wrap Up

    The Kettlebell community is becoming more popular. There's a lot of misinformation out there. I put this book out so some competent information would be available. When you go online, and look at some of the forms none of the messaging is correct. It's all rather vague, and sometimes over-inflated. Can you expect real results with the Kettle bell? Of course! Just don't expect these over-inflated results that you've been hearing about online. It's true that the kettlebell burns 1200 calories an hour. This means you can burn a pound of fat in 3 days if you do an hour everyday. That is an undeniable benefit of the Kettlebell. The problem is people don't tell you that you have to up the weight. They also don't include all these different variations of exercise. The Kettlebell is a core concentrated tool. With a powerful core you can use the Kettlebell in a number of ways. As long as you're willing to put in the effort you'll gain results. If you're trying to lose weight pick a kettlebell that's the right size for you. If you're trying to gain muscle than you need a kettlebell that weighs more. In my opinion if you have a friend, or a partner to do this kind of exercise with it really makes it easy. Every single day me, and my girlfriend who is now my wife would workout with kettlebells. Doing this together really helped us both stay focus. Try to partner up with one person or even a group of people it really makes it easier. Stick to the diet it will increase your energy. Stay consistent, and enjoy yourself. With that I bid you farewell. I'm the Workout King have a great life, and great health.

www.ingramcontent.com/pod-product-compliance
Lightning Source LLC
Chambersburg PA
CBHW062115280526
45788CB00003B/1475